CASE
MANAGEMENT
A PALLIATIVE
PERSPECTIVE

RHODA NEADER RN, CHPN, CCM

outskirts
press

Outskirts Press, Inc.
http://www.outskirtspress.com

ISBN: 978-1-4787-5215-8

Outskirts Press and the "OP" logo are trademarks belonging to Outskirts Press, Inc.

PRINTED IN THE UNITED STATES OF AMERICA

Table of Contents

Introduction

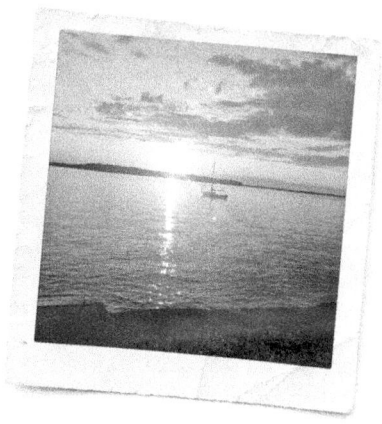

The contents of this book represent a minute slice of my years in nursing, hospice and palliative care as well as with case management. The situations are real. However there is no information to reveal the patient, demographics, or any situation that might compromise an individual patient's confidentiality.

At an ethics seminar that I attended, the general discussion after was one of significant lack of knowledge in the role of the case manager, palliative care and clinical ethics. There have been many individuals in my life that have an extensive knowledge base, and I am by no means an expert on any or one subject. I felt it might be useful to share my clinical practice role, what I feel could play an expanded role in many areas of case management, and truly more holistically support the patient populations that we serve.

I would like to acknowledge:
My husband John who supports me in many ways
Our children, who are finding their own paths in life.
Diana Peirce, hospice director, mentor and friend who led us all by example
My colleagues, friends and family

Case Management and the Evolution That Leads Many Nurses to It

> *"I don't know what your destiny will be, but one thing I do know: the only ones among you who will be truly really happy are those who have sought and found how to serve."*
>
> ALBERT SCHWITZER

The role of the case manager has taken many shapes and forms over the past few years. Workers comp case managers, home health and hospice case managers and insurance case managers are evolving and growing. It is no wonder why patients find case managers so beneficial with the ever changing health care situation and the complex maze that they have to maneuver.

My beginning story is like so many of ours. I started as a hospital floor nurse. I remember we would always stand for the physician to give him or her our chair. The patient usually never questioned the treatment plan that was offered. Stem cell replacements were unheard of. Bone marrow transplants were a huge undertaking. Heart and kidney transplants were not done yet. TPN (Total Parental Nutrition) was new in the hospitals. Nurses wore expensive, easily soiled white uniforms, white and easily torn stockings, and white shoes that we were expected to keep very clean. We had those little white caps and pins. Each patient was given a sponge bath along with a back rub every night. They were given a complete bath with a linen change every morning, and if the patient was unable to feed himself, we would sit and feed him. Medications were poured from a little med room. Nurses used to smoke in the little room and give a verbal report for shift change. Nursing unions were unheard of. I started working as a graduate nurse for $3.91/ hour. Yes, really.

Later, I was a director of nursing in a little nursing home in rural Vermont. I then went to a rural community home health agency (VNA), where I met the most fabulous hospice director, Diana Pierce. I fell in love with hospice (there was no palliative care back then) and it has been my love and passion for the years following. There was no Medicare hospice benefit back then. Many small home hospices in the state were pretty shaky. There was only six of us on the original hospice team and we often covered a hundred or more miles daily, walked into many snow filled drives, carried supplies and necessary things, including a loaf of bread, on the way. The hospice team was very tight knit, loving and supportive. When our dog, "Smokey" died (a dog I was asked to take after his owner died in hospice), we had a little candle light ceremony with a ship going out to sea, with my children and the hospice team.

I got many of my cooking recipes from my hospice families. They would have me taste this or that, then they would hurry off to copy it. Some families had no central heat. Some had no running water. Some were very poor. I found that they were very loving and very devoted to each other and to their hospice nurses. They were glorious days. Many of the same dear people are still on the team, still driving, still working the long days into the nights, and supporting the patients and each other.

We would often meet our unfortunate hospice patients as they were nearing death. It was not uncommon to meet a patient who was experiencing a fecal impaction, on opioids and not on a bowel program. We would make the best of it. It was the beginnings that made the wonderful unforgettable bonds and memories that still brings a smile to my face. We would sometimes just be together with a dying family member, talking, singing, or just sitting in quiet.

Sometime, early on, our Diana got Medicare certification for our hospice. We got paid, and it was a really big deal. Before I knew it, the 25 employee agency was 400 plus.

The palliative care patients were in higher numbers. We had more hospice nurses, wonderful nurse's aides, a full time social worker and a full interdisciplinary team. The local oncology office and nurse practitioner, along with the physicians, grew to respect us and the program blossomed. Patients died in comfort and dignity in their homes with families resting nearby.

I went on to work at Blue Cross Blue Shield of Vermont (BCBSVT) and was fortunate to develop the palliative/ hospice case management program. There were specialty case managers, innovative medical directors, and great case management support staff. The Blue Cross Blue Shield of Vermont case management program won national awards. Sometimes I would go out to meet our patients and the palliative / hospice nurses. I would, at times, companion people all over the country.

I went on to work at The University of Vermont Medical Center which is a 500 bed tertiary hospital in northwestern Vermont. This was a start-up hospital case management program and I worked as an oncology and end of life case manager. Each case manager was assigned to specific physician or physician group. I followed the University oncology group and another private oncology group. I confess that I saw myself as a palliative care nurse as well as a case manager. The pace was fast and furious, but the case manager role came to be appreciated.

We followed our patients and families from point of entry into the hospital, throughout their stay, and back out into the community. We were indeed fortunate in Vermont. We had the strong work ethic of the nurses, the evolving case management program, and the collaboration of our colleagues within and outside the hospital. In upstate NY, our neighboring state, and in Vermont, many of the case managers, nurses, home health and hospice nurses, and insurance case managers know and respect each other. We case managers acted as patient advocates and coordinators of care by getting approval to authorize the inpatient stays. We referred services, got prior approvals for meds, etc. and kept the plates in the air most of the time.

The winters in Vermont are sometimes as low as -30 degrees and the snow can be one to two feet at a snowfall. This can make commuting for patients and families very taxing. Many patients came for care from greater than 3 hours away that live in upstate NY.

The mountains are beautiful and the air is crisp and clean. In the spring, the back roads can be so muddy that you have to "ride the ridges" early in the morning while the ground is partially frozen and firm, or you can sink right in. Many a car or school bus would get stuck in the mud. I remember going out in the spring with a JCAHO surveyor when I was working in hospice. We couldn't get to the home, so we had to go to another town on the blacktop road and come up over an alternative route. She couldn't believe it! In Vermont the summer is green, green, green. The falls are beautiful, with foliage all around, people picking apples, pumpkins in the field, and folks preparing for winter. The people are kind, honest, and trusting, so unlike many other places. An oncology patient may often travel up to 60 or more miles to receive radiation. Radiation therapy can be daily for up to 4-6 weeks. Transportation needs were often complex and problematic.

Vermont did not have competing home health agencies/ palliative care and hospices. It was one agency that can cover greater than a 50 mile radius. Northern Vermont had a blossoming palliative community program. They were part of the Robert Wood Johnson Foundation movement, where the goal was for more than 50% of the physicians to make home visits on their palliative/ hospice patients. Folks come into the homes playing guitars, or quietly listening, singing, crying or laughing at a touching story or moment.

Case management has evolved, as have nurses, social workers and the health care system. We no longer stand for the physician when he or she enters a nursing unit like we used to. We often call them by their first name. We grew to love our bright caring residents from UVM and our physicians, our floor nurses and our patients. We have a role in the midst of it all, helping our patients navigate thought their stay and transition out of the hospital setting.

The inpatient case manager has the benefit of the one on one with the patient and/or family. It may be the best opportunity to assess barriers, strengths and needs. The insurance or telephonic case manager does not always have the additional sensory input when talking with the patient/ family. However, I have found that a great deal of trust, support and advocacy can be achieved. When you only have the telephone to communicate, the interview and listening skills are highly tuned. Also, the patient may relay to the telephonic case manager many things that they might not tell others. The community case manager has the opportunity to see the patient in their environment. They may be more relaxed and trusting with the continuity of "their" case manager. This case manager may also be tuned into many things that others may not have known. Good communication and collaboration is always optimal with our colleagues, and should not be overlooked for the overall well-being of the patient. The CMSA (Case Management Society of America) has become a sophisticated foundation for those of us in case management. The leaders are strong, highly intelligent, and assertive with enormous knowledge bases. There are standards of practice for case managers that I would strongly recommend all to read. This is one avenue for the case manager to become certified and remain enlightened and informed.

"If you help others, you will be helped:
perhaps tomorrow, perhaps in one hundred
years, but you will be helped"

G.I GURDJIEFF

THE CODE THAT I STRIVE FOR IS:

- Advocacy above all else
- Encourage autonomy
- Do good
- Do no harm
- Communicate
- Collaborate
- Refer
- Companion
- Listen- It can be the single most important thing that you do.

Palliative Care and its Role in Case Management

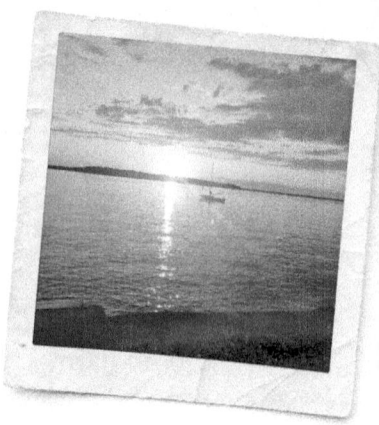

CHAPTER 2

What exactly is palliative care? Many of you might think. "What does that have to do with case management?"

Whether it is the fast pace of the case manager within the in-patient setting, the community setting, or for the insurance based case manager, palliative care has a vital role for our patients and families.

"Palliative care is the comprehensive management of patients' physical, psychological, social, spiritual, and existential needs. It is especially suited to the care of people with incurable, progressive illnesses".[1]

IN 2000 THE AMERICAN BOARD OF HOSPICE AND PALLIATIVE MEDICINE SAID PALLIATIVE MEDICINE IS:

"The medical discipline of the broad therapeutic model is known as palliative care. This discipline and model of care are devoted to achieve the best possible quality of life of the patient and family

---

1   *Last Acts 1997*

throughout the course of a life-threatening illness, through the relief of suffering, and the control of symptoms. Such relief requires the comprehensive assessment and interdisciplinary team management of the physical, psychological, social and spiritual needs of patients and their families. Palliative medicine helps the patient and family face the prospect of death assured that comfort will be a priority, values and decisions will be respected, spiritual and psycholosocial needs will be addressed, practical support will be available, and opportunities will exist for growth and resolution."

So, what is the difference between palliative care and hospice care? They seem so alike and sometimes used interchangeably. One might say, "This patient is just getting chemo and radiation and they are young. Yes, they may have advanced disease and lesions but they are not dying."

Most professionals would agree that any individual that has metastatic disease would be best taken care of with palliative treatment. The patient's goal may be to keep the disease at bay, or hold out for a remission or cure. They may undergo treatment with TPN, radiation, chemotherapy, or transfusions. A priority needs to be maximizing the quality of life for that individual for as long as they are alive, regardless of the time. Basically, anyone with an advanced disease would benefit from the holistic palliative approach. This is regardless of whether they are getting treatment or not.

I love the way the ethicist said it in a conference, pointing to a graph: *"Before palliative care, individuals were treated, treated, treated, treated, then oops... death. Then they were treated, treated, treated, perhaps palliative care...and maybe a transition to hospice... then death with companioning and support."*

FOR INDIVIDUALS TO BE ELIGIBLE FOR HOSPICE THEY MUST:

1. Have exhausted all treatment options

The exception for some private insurance is occasionally allowing TPN, transfusions, or high dollar drugs that would contribute to quality of life. This is particularly the case is the patient is trying to reach a goal of a special event, etc.

Medicare would allow medications to manage pain and symptoms, DME (durable medical equipment), hospice interdiciplinary staff, E.G. medical director, nurse, social worker, pastoral care, grief counselors, liscensed nurses aides and volunteers.

2. Make a commitment to have pain and symptoms managed at home or a hospice inpatient setting

The hospice interdisciplinary team (IDT), patient of family would have set up a plan of care, established goals, and have an "emergency" plan. The family has a 24 hour number to call, which can be for counseling over the phone, or to set up a visit from the nurse, physician or NP to visit the home.

On rare occasions, the patient is placed in a hospice inpatient setting for an acute situation, such as symptom management or respite.

3. Have a limited life expectancy of 6 months or less.

This may be difficult, as each individual is different.

Effective pain and symptom management often offers good quality time, so this is generally thought of as having "a short time to live".

The non-oncology patient is sometimes overlooked. The patients with end-stage COPD, end-stage cardiac disease, Parkinson's disease, or neurological disease may be overlooked. Generally patients with progressive deterioration over the previous 12 months may be eligible for hospice.

When addressing this option with a patient or family it is important to consider the patient or family understanding of the disease. If appropriate, it can often mean a much richer benefit for the patient to access the hospice benefit. If the goal is not to be managed in the hospice setting, then palliative care is a more appropriate option. Hospice patients do not have to be homebound, which is important to relay to the patient/ family.

"The family physician, by virtue of unique training and experience, is in a position to provide a leadership role in the hospice movement.

The concept of hospice is one of comprehensive care for the dying. The physical facilities may be very extensive or quite minimal. The AAFP, therefore, chooses to define hospice in terms of of what it does rather than the institution in which it is performed.

A hospice is a program designed to care for the dying, and their special needs. Among these services all hospice programs should include:

a. *Control of pain and other symptoms through medication, environmental adjustment, and education.*
b. *Psychosocial support for both the patient and family, including all phases from diagnosis though bereavement.*
c. *Medical services commensurate with the needs of the patient*
d. *Interdiciplinary "team" approach to patient care, patient and family support, and education with physician leadership.*
e. *Integration into existing facilities where possible.*
f. *Specially trained personnel with expertise in care of the dying and their families."[2]*

ANOTHER DEFINITION OF HOSPICE

"Hospice [care]= Support and care for the person in the last phase of an incurable disease so that they may live as fully and comfortably as possible.

Hospice [care]:

- *recognizes that the dying process is a part of the normal process of living and focuses on enhancing the quality of remaining life.*
- *affirms life and neither hastens nor postpones death.*
- *exists in the hope and belief that through appropriate care, and the promotion of caring community sensitive to their needs, that individuals and their families may be free to attain a degree of satisfaction in preparation for death.*
- *recognizes that human growth and development can be a life-long process*

---

2   (1979) (2002) Copyright 2004, American Academy of Family Physicians

- *seeks to preserve and promote the inherent potential for growth within individuals and families during the last phase of life.*
- *Offers palliative care for all individuals and their families without regard to age, gender, nationality, race, creed, sexual orientation, disability, diagnosis, availability of a primary care provider, or ability to pay.*

  Hospice programs provide state of the art palliative care and supportive services to the individuals as the end of their lives, their family members and significant others. 24 hours a day, seven days a week, in both the home and facility-based settings. Physical,, social, spiritual, and emotional care is provided by clinically-directed interdisciplinary team

  Consisting of patient and their families, professionals and volunteers during the:

  Last stages of an illness;
  Dying process; and
  Bereavement period.[3]

So one might say, "What does all this have to do with me? I am very busy. I don't have time for all this palliative care stuff. One might also feel that it should be up to the physician". Or "My job is to get the patient through the system as best as I can. I am not a hospice nurse."

In the role of case manager we are often the one person the patient consistently sees. The one that touches their inside world and can connect them to the outside world after they leave the

---

3   Hospice Standards of Practice, National Hospice and Palliative Care Organization<http://www. nhpnco.org>. 2000

hospital. In just one brief assessment, it can often become very evident what the physical, cultural and ethical needs are for this patient and/or family. What better advocate for this patient than the case manager?

We should be ascertaining from the patient, team, and/or family what those needs are. Are they being met? What barriers are there to meeting them? This does in no way mean that we are the "be all, end all." It simply means that we are the coordinator, the facilitator and the referral person to help accomplish this when and if this is the patient's choice.

> *"My goal was to break through the layer of professional denial that prohibited patients from airing their inner-most concerns."*
>
> Elizabeth Kubler-Ross,
> *On Death and Dying,* 1969

CASE MANAGEMENT AND/OR PALLIATIVE NEEDS TO BE ADDRESSED:

- **Physical needs**
- **Emotional needs**
- **Psycho/Social needs**
- **Spiritual needs**
- **Cultural needs**
- **Ethical needs**

PHYSICAL NEEDS

Pain- *"An unpleasant subjective sensory and emotional experience associated with actual or potential tissue damage or described in terms of such damage."*[4]

The Hospice and Palliative Nurses Association (HPNA) supports the provision of appropriate pain management for patients in all clinical settings. It is the position of HPNA Board of Directors that:

- All health care providers have the obligation to all people, including vulnerable populations such as infants, children, and the elderly, facing progressive, life–limiting illness, have the right to optimal pain relief.
- Believe the patient's report of pain.
- Pain assessment and management should incorporate principles of cultural sensitivity as well as patients' values and beliefs.
- All healthcare professionals caring for patients with progressive, life-threatening illness need to acquire and utilize current knowledge and skills to implement appropriate pain management.
- Healthcare organizations need to adopt policies and procedures that address the assessment, pharmacologic, and non-pharmacologic management of pain.
- Pain management should include, as appropriate, advanced technology.
- Pain assessments and management should be aligned with

---

4   American Pain Society, Principles of Analgesic Use in the Treatment of Acute Pain and Cancer Pain. 4th ed. Glenview, Ill. Author: 1999

evidence-based practice.

- The need for regulatory control of opioids must be balanced with access to opioids for all patients who need them.
- Pain management should be part of education for all healthcare providers who are caring for patients with advanced, life-limiting illness.
- Healthcare professionals must advocate for their patients to ensure adequate pain relief.
- Uncontrolled pain should be considered an emergency, with all healthcare professionals taking responsibility to provide relief.
- Patients have the right to participate actively in decisions about their pain management.
- Families should be supported in their efforts to observe and relieve pain when appropriate
- Hospice and palliative care programs should share their knowledge of pain management concepts with others in their communities.
- Use of placebos for pain management is inappropriate."[5]

Pain can sometimes be difficult to detect. Chronic pain may be present despite an individual talking, laughing, or walking. They may have been living with pain for quite some time, may be depressed, or distant. Ask them to describe the pain and what makes it better or worse. Clarify that the scale that you are using is the one that your facility or agency is using and that it is the same for the patient.

I once met a patient that was sobbing and telling me that she

---

5   "Journal of Hospice and Palliative Nursing" Vol. 6, No. 1. January –March 2004

couldn't take the pain anymore. She had been rating her pain at 4. It was assumed that it was 4 on a 0-10 scale. However, it was a 4 on a 0-5 scale. Once this was identified it was relayed to the physician involved in her care and the patient was made comfortable.

An inpatient palliative clinician or team is an excellent resource if you are fortunate enough to have one. Many hospitals have contracts with local palliative / hospice physicians or teams. Never assume that a patient is comfortable, always ask. You should also talk with the nurses providing care, as they are a wealth of information. If nothing is ordered, advocate for the patient by following up. Follow-up and advocate either with the nurse, the physician, or recommend a pain consult if available. A case manager should always be an advocate for our patients.

Physical needs may or may not be pain. Respiratory distress, agitation, constipation, nausea and vomiting also need to be addressed. Using the same scale as the pain scale often helps to quantify the symptom. It is important for the patient to understand that symptom management should be a priority and right.

EMOTIONAL NEEDS

Emotional needs can run amuck in a crisis setting. Patients and families can become distraught, angry; they may shift blame, and generally just feel angry and overwhelmed by the circumstances. As you become more seasoned as a case manager, it somehow becomes less personal when this happens. I have personally had a door or two slammed in my face, or an angry outburst or two. As I have gotten more experienced, it somehow seems to be a lot less personal. If not taken personally, the patient or family will often feel validated and supported. Apologies and reassurance that it isn't taken personally are appreciated. This may be an opportunity for a referral to our social work colleagues for additional patient and family support.

Abuse from patients and families is not ok. If this is problematic, report this to your supervisor for assistance in handling the situation. Abuse of the elderly, child or spousal abuse, or any other abuse needs to be reported to your social worker colleagues, or whatever administrative channel that is within your policy.

PHYCHOSOCIAL NEEDS

This can often be a difficult time for patients and families, especially if the patient if young and facing months of treatment or rehabilitation, struggling financially, trying to hold a job, etc. It is advantageous to make referrals as accepted by the patient to agencies, to pediatric or adult social workers, support groups, grief counselors, and/ or any referral options that would be appropriate.

SPIRITUAL NEEDS

A worker in pastoral care in my former tertiary hospital told me that he was unable to support the patient with his spiritual needs because the patient was in so much physical pain that it consumed all of his energy. Overwhelmed, his goal was primarily relief of pain and symptoms before any spiritual needs could even be addressed. Case in point, it is virtually impossible to establish the holistic needs of the patient if the basic pain and symptom management needs are not managed.

Spiritual needs are not the same as religious needs. I used to love it the way that my hospice agency staff would ask the patient,

"What is the source of your spiritual support?" The source of their support may be a newly born grandchild, being on their back porch listening to the brook or to birds, or being with family or loved ones. It may be a very personal one on one relationship with their higher power, an affiliation with their synagogue or parish, or they may have no belief system at all.

It is important to recognize if there is a need, and to facilitate a referral if needed. Most pastoral care providers can be nondenominational, may refer to the patient's own clergy, or simply support the patient and/or family though a crisis.

It is always important to keep in mind that the patient's belief system is their belief system, not ours. It is highly inappropriate to attempt any influence on the patient or family using our perceptions of what we think that they need.

CULTURAL NEEDS

More and more we need to become aware of diversity. We need to be mindful of the individual's cultural and ethnic needs. I once had a patient that was Filipino. I researched that the adult Filipino will often delegate any health care decisions to their eldest child, who in this case, was outside the US. In their culture, they often do not want to appear impolite, so they may nod yes when they might like to challenge or disagree with an opinion. In this case, I asked the patient if I could talk to the eldest daughter. He and his wife readily agreed. The daughter then discussed options with her parents, and a discharge plan that was very different from what I might had thought best was chosen. Weeks later I received a letter of appreciation from the spouse and daughter. We had researched the potential cultural needs, made copies for the accepting facility and hospice, and passed on the necessary information to meet this patient's and family's cultural needs.

Take a moment to research any potential cultural needs, then document and relay the information to other caregivers outside of the family unit. It will help to ensure respect and dignity.

ETHICAL NEEDS

We all have seen and heard of ethical dilemmas over the years. It is important to establish early on in your relationship with your patient and your patient's family that their wishes need to be communicated, and subsequently put into writing. If the patient is within the inpatient setting, any limitations of care should be established and documented in a clear visible place to all caregivers.

Life planning, durable power of attorney for healthcare (DPOAHC), or sometimes now called advanced care planning, is an informed decision making process that should take place after a lot of thought and communication. I recommend completing it when the patient and family are most rested, have worked through the "grey areas", and have had an open conversation with any pertinent family or friends that should be included in a decision making capacity. I usually offer the booklet with instructions then go over it carefully with the patient and family. I usually give copies to the partner/ spouse/ family of the actual form to take home to discuss (if they need it) and to complete if they choose. Many patients and families are now computer savvy and can download the appropriate forms with instructions.

Advanced directives may vary from state to state, and is only in the event that the individual cannot speak for himself. It can be revised at any time. It is important, however, that the signing is witnessed by two impartial individuals of legal age or a notary. It cannot be the DPOAHC, the nurse or anyone that could be perceived as influencing care.

"Goals of care must be established before one can deliberate the benefits or burdens of a particular treatment. Planning interventions without regard to the goals of care may be the source of ethical conflict. Goals of care must be determined collaboratively with the patient and family, the physician, the nurse, and other team members, facilitating decisions through effective communication and deliberation. For example, the patient cannot truly give informed consent without knowing the potential outcomes of proposed interventions based on his or her individual diagnosis and prognosis."[6]

In many hospitals and agencies there is an ethicist that can be of benefit if this is unclear. The patient and/or family must ok things first, and discuss with the physician if this cannot be established. The can be offered to the patient and/or family, the physician, or the team. It is always in the best interest of the patient to consult an ethicist if there is any doubt, as it can greatly relieve the family's stress and burden, and identify what would be in the patient's best interest if he or she cannot speak for himself or herself.

---

6   "Journal of Hospice and Palliative Nursing" Vol 6, NO1. January-March 2004

COMFORT CARE SHOULD IT BE
ONLY FOR THE DYING?

Comfort:[7]

To soothe in time of affliction or distress.

To ease physically: relieve

To make strong; to invigorate; to fortify; to corroborate. [Obs]—Wyclif.

To impart strength and hope to; to encourage/ to relieve; to console; to cheer.

> *"The moment one gives a close attention to anything, even a blade of grass, it becomes a mysterious, awesome, indescribably magnificent world in itself"*
>
> HENRY MILLER

As nurses, we all try to comfort our patients. As the years pass, technology has significantly increased, care needs have become more complex, documentation more comprehensive, and nursing care is more demanding. Where is there time to give comfort, you might ask? Patients diagnosed with a new metastatic disease, a short time to live, or who have reached the end stage of a chronic debilitating disease needs support early on.

Comfort is given in many shapes and forms. It can be done by simply sitting or actively listening. An elderly nun once told me, if you can't do anything at all, try to turn the patient's pillow to make it feel a little fresher for them. So many times when I see

---

7   Webster's Revised Unabridged Dictionary, C 1996, 1998 MICRA, Inc

a patient, offering comfort may not be doing any big thing. It may be just being present in the moment with that individual. I look back at the evolution of nursing, back to when all patients received baths, backrubs, lotion rubs, and I miss that. Times are fast paced for the bedside nurses today. So much is focused on the great tasks at hand, and there may not be enough hours in the day. How can we give comfort in this busy world?

TO SOOTH IN TIME OF AFFLICTION OR DISTRESS

Once I helped a widower with some bills that he was receiving after the death of his wife. He had a small child, his wife's employer had switched insurance companies, and after her death he began getting bills. Many bills were duplicates, with amounts that he found confusing. He told me that he had spent over fifteen hours in one week trying to sort it all out. He also shared that he had "called and called" to get answers but was unable to make any progress with it. Unfortunately, this is not uncommon. He asked me if there was anything that I could do to help. I told him that I would try to take a look at it and perhaps ask for the help of my social worker to help us. He began to explain the charges, and had written little edit notes beside the costs associated with the procedure. It was becoming more and more evident that he was reliving the last few weeks, days, and hours, and had totally broken down in grief. He was a strong man who was grieving appropriately. He and his son were getting support, but he needed to tell how those events made him feel. Retelling the story helps get out and process the grief. I could only listen. My helping him with the bills was a piece of it, but listening to him tell of his love, his sadness, regrets, and his loss was what he really needed. He told me that he had never cried in all those weeks when his wife was becoming more ill, going into palliative care, in and out of the hospital, and now he could.

What I learned and what he gave to me was far more than the helping with the bills. I saw a glimpse into the life of a beautiful couple. I saw their courage, trust, love, and strength.

TO EASE PHYSICALLY; RELIEVE

How many times have you visited a patient to have them tell you that their pain is perhaps a 5 out of 10? You look at them and they are a third down the bed and their pillow cases are half off. They are on the plastic part of the pillow and generally in a disarray. Medication may be warranted, but how often are simple things overlooked? For example, the rubbing, the fluffing, the moistening of the lips, a fresh drink, a touch, a smile. Of all the things that I feel that have been most lost over the years in nursing, this is one of the most important. I wish somehow that it could be brought back into our culture, the basic core of nursing.

TO MAKE STRONG; TO INVIGORATE; TO FORTIFY; TO CORROBORATE. [OBS.]-WYCLIF.

I love this aspect of comfort. Have you ever noticed the difference between a severely debilitated individual who is feeling powerless and that same person when they become empowered? This is a visible difference. Even the most severely ill can be empowered by making as many choices as they can for themselves-for their care; their life; their thoughts; and their goals. When the patient trusts that he/ she is in the driving seat of his or her care their entire affect changes. They may be sad, grieving, or angry, but they are fortified. Try to encourage this. Be honest, kind, and empowering.

TO IMPART STRENGTH AND HOPE TO; TO ENCOURAGE; TO RELIEVE; TO CONSOLE; TO CHEER.

I think that most of us would agree that even in hospice, we never want to take away hope. Hope takes many forms. There is hope of remission, or slowing of disease. There is hope of resolution with self or loved ones. There is the hope of being functional as long as possible, of being loved and respected, and also the hope of being companioned until death. Hope is a beautiful thing to always remember.

"The natural lights of the human mind are not from pleasure to pleasure, but from hope to hope."
SAMUAL JOHNSON

Finally, always offer our local palliative care and /or hospice agency for additional support. As my hospice director once said, "They are a diamond in your community."

Clarifying the Patient's Goal

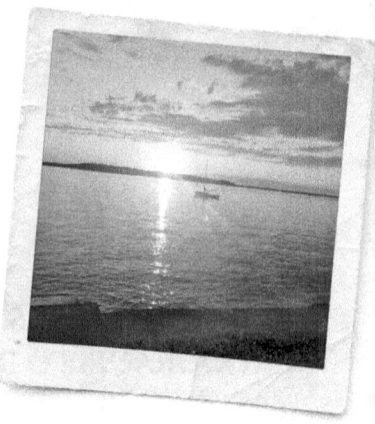

CHAPTER 3

*"I live in a very small house, but my
windows look out on a very large world."*

CONFUCIUS

I find that clarifying the patient's goals has to be one of the most essential parts of the case manager's assessment. You can't and shouldn't assume that what you are reading in the clinical record or what you are hearing is really what the patient's actual goal is. Always ask what his or her goal is, as it is vital to the discharge plan. As a true patient advocate, we need to be absolutely clear what it is that they would like to accomplish. But what if that is too uncomfortable, or is not a reasonable goal? Try to find out, perhaps by breaking it down into pieces, and go from there.

*"God allows us to experience the low
points of life in order to teach us lessons
we could not learn in any other way."*

C.S. Lewis

I have never forgotten what a woman told me years ago. She was a young, highly functioning woman who thought what she had was an acute illness. She was admitted to a hospital, and was found to have metastatic disease with no viable treatment options to offer her. The report was that she must have had an underlying, undiagnosed psychiatric disorder. She was literally placed in a "strait jacket" for what was perceived as an acute psychotic event, and eventually discharged home with home hospice services. When I first met her she told me her story, pouring out her heart. At the end of our visit she said to me, "You are the first person that has actually asked me what I wanted. There were dozens of medical people around me, doing this, saying that, but no one asked me what I wanted or needed. I just lost it and totally shut down."

Another young man with a long struggle with lymphoma was in the hospital for what was initially days, then weeks, then months. He and his wife had two high school age children. His family would visit as they could. They lived over two hours away. He was in and out of the intensive care and transfusion dependent. He became depressed, despondent, weak, and very lonely. I felt that I needed to sit with him and find out what his goal was. I didn't want to supersede what his physicians and team were trying to do. He was not noted to be terminal, but he was not getting any better and he was slipping into a worsening condition. When I met with him and his wife, I asked them what they wanted. He clearly told me, "I want to go home, I am tired of all this." After discussing what the outcomes would be and how it could be accomplished. I advised the team and a discharge date was set. Home hospice was set up along with the medications, equipment, and potential needs relayed. I called this patient a week later. We had sent him to his summer camp as was his wish. His wife said, "It was quite a ride... The road was pretty rough going into camp, with grass growing in the middle of the road, but the ambulance just kept climbing the hill into camp to get him home."

I then spoke with the patient. He said to me, "Thank you so much for helping me. I am looking out over the lake, it is so beautiful... my family and friends are here, and I am so happy. I just want you to know that."

*"Let us be like a bird for a moment perched
On a frail branch while he sings;
Though he feels it bend, yet he sings his song,
Knowing he has wings"*

VICTOR HUGO

I remember when I first came to that hospital as a case manager. I was reviewing the chart of an elderly man who was in the intensive care unit with recurrent respiratory failure. He was already intubated. I found that he had had 16 admissions already that year: to either the emergency room, in house as outpatient observation, or usually as inpatient with long length of stays. He had had more than a few of these admissions to the intensive care unit. He had gone home two days earlier but was again readmitted. When I read the admission note, I found that it was noted that he had not picked up his antibiotic or his prednisone when he was last discharged.

He had become increasing short of breath, his health spiraled downward, and he was readmitted back to the hospital. I met with his wife, found that they "didn't need home health" and continued to follow him daily. When the patient was weaned off the ventilator and transferred to the medical floor, I met with him and his wife, and eventually with this grown children.

He stated that his goal was to go home, that he didn't need any help, and brushed me off. I gently reintroduced the idea of home health (at minimum) if his goal was to remain at home. He agreed. I set up a plan with the home health to follow him at home to establish medication adherence and assess his cardiopulmonary status. Two weeks later, he was readmitted with pneumonia. He had reportedly refused to have home health services when the nurse came to the home. I met with him again to gently reestablish his goal of remaining at home, and find a way that it might be accomplished.

"I know that I should have never sent them away. They would have helped me." he said. There was an inroad into what he wanted, and what he wanted to accomplish. Eventually he was readmitted again with respiratory failure simply because of disease progression. After clarifying with the physician and meeting again with the patient, family, and medical team, we gently addressed the issue of his disease progression. I cannot emphasize this enough. It is very important to not only have the correct clinical picture, but to have an understanding of the progression that the disease may take. The long and the short of it is that this elderly, gruff, non-adhering man came up with a plan with his physician and family. He decided that if he were to be on a ventilator again for end stage respiratory failure that he would only want to be on a ventilator for seven days. Eventually this did indeed happen, and his life support was withdrawn as was his wish He died peacefully surrounded by his family.

"If you want to lift yourself up,
lift up someone else."
BOOKER T. WASHINGTON

Years ago I remember meeting a man who had just been admitted to hospice. He had metastatic gastric cancer. He had never had palliative care, home care, or any other community supports. He was angry, cachectic, in significant pain, and was spending his days and nights in a recliner. He and his wife told me his story, and he eventually told me what his worst fear was.

"The doctor told me that I wasn't going to die of cancer, but I was going to starve to death." We discussed what the natural progression of his disease would look like, what options he could be offered for pain and symptom management, and how his last few weeks could be very different. He was soon pain free; able to walk and say his good byes, and to have energy left to come to terms with his dying process. He was finally able to address his concerns for leaving his wife behind. He left her many household tips, advice and instructions. I grew to love them both. The one thing that I always try to discuss is what they want. I would tell my patients that we would do it their way right from the start. Once this is established, the patient feels that he or she has some control, won't be powerless, and that things won't be done that he or she doesn't want.

One night I was called out after being told that this same patient was actively dying. When I entered the house, the family was all there and his wife was sitting beside him, holding his hand. He was unresponsive and had been for several hours. His breathing was irregular and he was moribund. She asked me to come over, and I sat there holding his other hand. I said quietly, "I am so glad that he did it his way, and he looks so beautiful." He quickly took his arms, one from each of us on each side of his bed, and he put his hands on the side of our faces for a brief moment. It was absolutely touching.

"The most beautiful thing that we can experience is the miraculous."
ALBERT EINSTEIN

What if the patient's or family's goal seems totally unrealistic? Some time ago I had a patient with CNS lymphoma. He had a long struggle, had been in the hospital for a long time, was debilitated, and was having cognition issues. His wife, who was his strong advocate, was angry and frustrated. She felt that the staff should not ask him to do things, they could just tell him, "OK, let's go. You have to get up and moving." He would just listen and participate she told us. Physical therapy told me that they were unable to motivate him, and nothing seemed to be working. The patient was losing ground; his wife was becoming more concerned and frustrated, and feeling increasingly angry.

At that point I called together the key people providing care in the hospital- the spouse who was his DPOAHC, (the patient did not want to participate), and an ethicist. An ethicist can be invaluable in a complex patient and/or family situation. Goals were addressed and established. How to accomplish this?

It was established that his primary goal was to be home with his newly born grandchild, but he could not process this into a short term goal of getting out of bed, eating, or drinking. The plan was then put into place. Each time a request was made of this patient to engage in an activity, it was phased into words reflecting his short term goal. Statements such as, "If you want to go home to see your granddaughter you need to get out of bed," were made. Pictures were placed very close to him. The care plan was updated, and methods were used to break the goal into immediate images for this patient. It worked!

A discharge date was set, services and equipment were set up at home, and several days later, this very same patient walked (with a walker) out of the hospital with his wife to go home.

"Any man who does not believe in miracles is not a realist."

DAVID BEN GURION

I once had a palliative care patient that was a young attorney with Lou Gehrig's disease, also known as Amyotrophic Lateral Sclerosis (ALS). He was referred to me because the household was reported to be volatile.

He was quickly losing the ability to speak, could no longer walk, and was going to have a feeding tube placed. I believe that all patients, and particularly those with neurological diseases, need to clarify goals, understand choices, as well as outcomes. During the initial assessment, it was clear that no life planning had been done. The patient was highly intelligent but was addressing each and every medical situation only as it came along. We carefully discussed what his understanding of his disease was, where he felt that he was at in the process, and what his goal was. "I want to be home. I have a four year old son, and I want to be with him." He replied. We discussed the "what if" plan. What if you could no longer breathe on your own, what would you like to have done? He told me "I haven't really given it a thought... I guess I want a ventilator. I don't want to die. I am too young." I asked him how his wife was coping, and what supports and family did he have in the area that could be rallied and stay with him over time. "My wife is pretty unraveled. She has to work. There is no one."

Over time we came up with a list of questions for this man and his wife to discuss with his physician. At that time it was not feasible to have home ventilation as he did not have the supports to accomplish this at home. The local rehabs could not accommodate a ventilator patient. It was evident that to really accomplish the goal, that all the choices and outcomes needed to be addressed in advance. I called the palliative care RN that was covering his area and relayed this to her, and contacted his physician (neurologist) to let him know what he might need to expect with their next visit (which was the next week). Eventually the patient came up with his own plan with his physician and hospice team. He chose to die at home. He did not choose to opt for a ventilator. He was prepared for what to expect in the event that he could no longer breathe on his own, and he died in comfort and dignity at home in hospice care.

One of the most poignant examples of listening to the patient and family happened many years ago. I met a man in his 40s named Albert. He was married to Mary and they had a young daughter. He had recently been diagnosed with Non-Small Cell

Lung Carcinoma (NSCLC). His disease had progressed and he was admitted with metastasis to the brain. His wife was at his bedside as much as possible. She was articulate and was a strong advocate for her husband. She told me that he had an enormous amount of guilt over the fact that he had a long history of smoking prior to his diagnosis. He received inpatient chemotherapy and radiation. He was alert and oriented but over time was no longer able to work and had become increasing deconditioned.

On his last admission to the hospital he had become increasingly short of breath. He was followed closely by his primary pulmonary oncologist. He had recurrent loculated pleural effusions and the thoracentesis to drain the fluid had become ineffective. He was apparently discharged home.

A few weeks later his wife came to see me at the hospital. She told me that Albert had died but shared with me the events leading up to his demise. I sat with her and she articulated that she could hear her husband "screaming in pain" as the team attempted to unsuccessfully drain fluid off his lungs. He was already on-service with palliative care and home oxygen and equipment were in place. What she told me next was that during all of Albert's treatments, admissions, and crisis situations, it had not "registered" that Albert was actually dying. She then went on to tell me that at the end of her husband's last hospital stay, the bedside nurse came from behind the curtain in the room and told her that Albert was dying. She told me that she was taken aback and was not really aware of this because they were always so focused on treatment and on Albert feeling better. She told me that if Albert and she had known this, weeks earlier that they would have spent the time differently and felt that they were robbed of that and that he suffered needlessly. I asked if she would like to meet with

Albert's oncologist and share her feelings with him and she told me that she would like that.

I have to say that I was not looking forward to a meeting. Who was I to put myself in this situation? I knew that I had to do it for Mary, so I set up the meeting. It was with Albert's wife, Mary, his oncologist and me. The three of us met in a small room. The relationship between Mary and Albert's oncologist was open and trusting. Mary began to articulate the events leading up to Albert's final days. She told Albert's oncologist that Albert was so weak that when she brought him home from the hospital that he crawled on his hands and knees to get to his bed. He was too weak to stand even with help. I was trying to be calm and supportive but actually I felt anxious inside. I tried to just be present in the moment. I watched as Mary went on to explain that had Albert known that he was dying, he would have made very different choices.

Albert's oncologist was directly across from Mary. He did not look away from her and he allowed her to get her story out without interruption. When she was finished he looked at her. He sincerely apologized for what Albert and she went through. He also told her that it would affect his oncology practice going forward.

Never doubt your ability that you are the patient's advocate, and that you have the ability to help clarify his or her goals. It cannot always be done quickly, nor can it always be done in a single session. It is a process that evolves as the patient can trust and believe that they are the focus of their care, not the system. Always remember that it is the patient's goal, not our goal.

Benefits and How to Make the Most of What You Have to Work with While Maximizing Options for Your Patient and Family

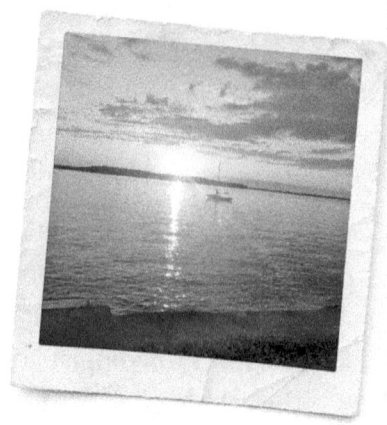

CHAPTER 4

"When you have lemons, make lemonade"
ANONYMOUS

We have all heard this phrase, but those of us in case management practice this each and every day. As medical care becomes more and more expensive, companies are paring costs for their employees. Patients are offered a multitude of treatment options that may extend life, but not necessarily give them quality of life. They frequently have to learn to navigate through the complexity of health care. Many patients do not have prescription coverage necessary for a long road of treatments that lie ahead, and there are still many individuals that have no insurance, that are not eligible, and may take weeks or months to access any healthcare benefit if at all. So what are we supposed to do with all that?

It is very important to find out from the patient and/or family that they understand their benefits. Does this person have prescription drug coverage? If patients need home infusion, do they have a benefit? Do they know what their home health, hospice, rehab or outpatient copays are? Sometimes the patient is too ill to discuss this, or may never have had to know. In this situation you have to verify on your own and offer choices.

Years ago I had a patient with metastatic disease in her fifties. She was married and lived in the neighboring state. She and her husband had no children. She was a hairdresser, and was the subscriber on her insurance policy. She had been admitted for a large pathological fracture and could not get out of bed. She and her husband had prided themselves on their ability to manage at home, to rely on each other, and their goal was for her to return home. Three issues were significant barriers to achieve this outcome. They had many friends, but none of their friends and family could be rallied to provide twenty four hour help. Getting out of bed in itself was problematic and the physical therapist working with the patient felt that rehab was key if the patient were to achieve the goal of returning safely to home. When checking the patient's benefits, and after many calls, it was clarified that the patient did not have any rehab benefit. The spouse was very upset, could not believe it, and continued to argue that something was very wrong. I clarified this with the supervisor of benefits at the patient's insurance company. I asked the spouse to bring in his copy of their insurance benefits. He met me the next morning saying, "I just can't believe that we were paying almost $600 a month and we don't even have a rehab benefit." So what to do next?

We called for a family team meeting with staff and physician's involved with the patient's care. We discussed benefits, options, and choice. The patient clearly did not want hospice as she was flying out of state to be evaluated for a clinical trial. Her state at that time did not have palliative care. They had separate home health agencies and hospice agencies. In a case like this, don't blame the insurance company case manager. Look at what you do have.

In this case, the patient had considerable savings. They were not wealthy by any means, but had some reserves. The option of self-paying at a sub-acute rehab was initiated and accepted. The rehab in their area was contracted with their insurance and the patient was accepted. The insurance case manager was able to "tweak" the benefit within the contract. There was not a way to get sub-acute rehab authorized and the patient did not meet the qualifications for acute rehab. However, the insurance case manager was able to adjust the home health benefit to allow for skilled nursing and physical therapy for what the patient would need when she transitioned home. At first the patient's spouse resisted this plan. He didn't want to spend any savings, and felt that he should have the rehab benefit. The reality is that they didn't. So sometimes it has to be brought back to the patient and family that this is the way it might be now. When their policy was up for renewal, I suggested that it might be wise to shop around for a more comprehensive policy. But sometimes you have to work with what you have.

It is always good to brainstorm with your colleagues. Collaboration is the key for the best possible outcome. The insurance case managers are doing their job, and they are the patient's advocate as well. I always offer the patient the option of getting an insurance case manager if it is available on their policy. It is so much better for the patient. The insurance case manager can sometimes come up with alternatives, and it is "one stop shopping" for the patient to set things up.

Case Management services are voluntary and the patients must give consent. If they understand the benefit, they rarely decline the additional support.

Always be aware of the medications that your patient is taking outside as well as might be discharging on from the hospital. For palliative care patients, there may be medications that can be very expensive, or may need prior approval. It is important to check in with them early on regarding what their prescription benefits are. You may have patients going home on enoxaparin with a coagulopathy and will need if for several weeks or months. They may likely need help. A significant number of oncology patients may have a coagulopathy impacting their disease and they may not have a prescription benefit. They may need prior approval or the medication exceeds the approved length of treatment.

They may be uninsured with a multitude of needs. They may not be willing or able to administer it, may not have had teaching, or have issues with adherence.

Brainstorm and network. What have you done in the past; and what could you do in this case? Do they have Medicaid? Could you get a voucher to cover the rest of the copayment? Can it be given in an outpatient clinic or physician's office? Do they qualify for an indigent program?

Take it a step at a time, offer the patient choices, and then proceed. Always share your wealth of knowledge with your colleagues. It will help your case management or social work department's collective knowledge base.

Some time ago I had an oncology patient that lived out of state. At that time many patients from upstate New York came to the University of Vermont Medical Center, as the area in which they lived was medically underserved at that time. This patient was married, they had no children, and she was elderly. She was admitted with a bacteremia, then developed pneumonia. She was going to need several weeks of IV antibiotics. She had Medicare primary and a "carve out" (often a retirement insurance that would stand on its own if no Medicare in place) secondary insurance with an infusion benefit. The home heath in her area did not have the staff or expertise to provide home infusion at that time. The home health agency could provide the PICC line care but not the IV infusion needs. The infusion company did not go out to the rural setting where the patient lived at that time. The community hospital was one half hour away, and did not have the expertise back then to manage the outpatient infusion pump needs. The patient was on 3 times a day IV antibiotic that could have safely been administered by a relatively simply IV push technique. However, the spouse could not perform this, and the patient also could not.

The patient's goal was to go home. She declined the sub-acute rehab and swing bed offer in her community hospital. She wanted to go home. So what did we do? We had the infusion vendor set up a programmed pump. The husband took her to the outpatient department of the community hospital. The infusion vendor met them at the hospital and taught the outpatient department management regarding the every 48 hours IV antibiotic cassette change. The home health agency provided the PICC line maintenance, and offered home nursing and physical therapy support. It was complex, but it was successful, and the patient was able to achieve her goal.

"I have closed the door on doubt.
I will go by what light I can find.
And hold up my hands
And reach them out."

IRENE PETIT MCKEEHAN

What if your patient has no insurance, they are under 65 years old, their disability has not gone through, and they need palliative and/or hospice care? This is not an uncommon theme for the case manager, but somehow the plan always seems to come together.

An important component of the initial assessment is not only the patient's age, demographics, and other key factors, but what is the insurance or payer information?

If the patient is over 65 and has only Original Medicare A with no other supplemental insurance, then prescriptions may be problematic. It is important to discuss with the patient and/ or family how they are paying for their prescriptions. Frequently it is a hardship for the patient. During the conversation, pay attention to any additional payer options. Would an individual have Medicaid options? (In some states called AHCCCS). If so, a discussion would open up other potential options. With anti-emetics costing $20 to $30 a pill or more, and long acting opioids costing as much if not more, it may be worth investigating.

The patient or family may have already exhausted any and all options. I always find it very beneficial to refer to my social work colleagues or patient financial services if available in your hospital for follow-up. If the patient is over resourced for Medicaid with long term chronic needs it warrants investigating long term

Medicaid options as early on as possible.

A case manager may be able to find the necessary medications through the pharmaceutical company indigent programs, or co-pay assistance programs. This may make a huge difference in pain and symptom management for the patient's adherence to taking the meds. The guidelines are usually very clear, and it might be worth looking in to. With no other supplemental insurance, the outpatient prescription may be problematic., During the conversation, pay attention to any additional payer options. Would the individual have Medicaid options? If so, a discussion would open up other potential options.

Original Medicare is a Federal benefit. However, it is not all encompassing. For an inpatient or hospital stay (considered a hospital, acute rehab or long term acute care hospital (LTAC) in 2018 the inpatient deductible and copayment is: $1,340 for each benefit period. Days 1-60: there no coinsurance for each benefit period. Days 61-90: $335 coinsurance for each benefit period. Days 91 and beyond: $670 coinsurance per each "lifetime" (can only be used once).[8]

---

8   http;//www.Medicare.gov

2018 costs at a glance	
Part A premium	Most people don't pay a monthly premium for Part A (sometimes called "premium-free Part A"). If you buy Part A, you'll pay up to $422 each month. If you paid Medicare taxes for less than 30 quarters, the standard Part A premium is $422. If you paid Medicare taxes for 30-39 quarters, the standard Part A premium is $232.
Part A hospital inpatient deductible and coinsurance	You pay: • $1,340 deductible for each benefit period • Days 1-60: $0 coinsurance for each benefit period • Days 61-90: $335 coinsurance per day of each benefit period • Days 91 and beyond: $670 coinsurance per each "lifetime reserve day" after day 90 for each benefit period (up to 60 days over your lifetime) • Beyond lifetime reserve days: all costs
Part B premium	The standard Part B premium amount is $134 (or higher depending on your income). However, some people who get Social Security benefits will pay less than this amount ($130 on average).
Part B deductible and coinsurance	$183 per year. After your deductible is met, you typically pay 20% of the Medicare-approved amount for most doctor services (including most doctor services while you're a hospital inpatient), outpatient therapy, and durable medical equipment.
Part C premium	The Part C monthly premium varies by plan. Compare costs for specific Part C plans.
Part D premium	The Part D monthly premium varies by plan (higher-income consumers may pay more). Compare costs for specific Part D plans.

For a skilled nursing facility (SNF/ subacute rehab) in most cases the patient requires an inpatient 3 day hospital qualifying stay within the 60 day benefit period to transition to SNF. The patient needs to meet the inpatient hospital criteria to qualify for a medically necessary SNF stay. Non-medically necessary hospital stays that do not qualify for hospital inpatient criteria do not qualify for SNF.[9]

Under Original Medicare, transitional care such as home health is covered under Medicare B. Deductibles and coinsurance applies. For home health services: skilled nursing visits (SN), physical Therapy (PT), occupational therapy (OT), home health aide (HHA), Medical Social Worker (MSW) there must be a skilled need. Custodial services are not a covered benefit under Original Medicare.

The cumulative total within the 60 inpatient days represents a benefit period. Many patients and families do not realize this. The Medicare patient must be out of the hospital or rehab setting for 60 consecutive days. For example if Mr. Doe was admitted to a community hospital, transferred to a tertiary center, then transferred to a higher specialty center, the 60 day inpatient days are the total of all the inpatient days. The copay is one-time copay for that benefit period. The facility usually keeps track of the total inpatient days. If a patient is nearing exhaustion of their inpatient days, they will often receive a letter. They may or may not understand, and families often are feeling overwhelmed. For extensive stays, if is helpful to keep this in mind.

Some patients do not have supplemental insurance, therefore would be billed the co pay days. Days 61-90 are those inpatient

9   Excerpt from: https://www.medicare.gov/your-medicare-costs/costs-at-a-glance/costs-at-glance.html

copay days. The copay per day is $335. Beyond the 90th day, the daily copay increases to $670. I like to think of it as a checking account, a savings account, and a retirement account. It might be advisable to opt for the secondary insurance to be converted to the primary payer. The secondary insurance would need to be a carve-out secondary insurance, or an insurance that would stand on it's on without Medicare. This would save the lifetime reserve days for a later time if needed for that patient. Note: A Medicare supplemental insurance would not be eligible to convert to the primary insurance.[10]

If the patient does not have supplemental insurance, then it is essential to plan for other options.

If the patient is discharged and remains out of the hospital inpatient setting and or the SNF, the acute rehab or the LTAC for the 60 day benefit period, the clock "resets" to the Original Medicare benefit again. (The exception would be the Original Medicare lifetime reserve days). If you have an extremely ill patient, and it is anticipated that they will have extensive needs it is best to relay this information to the patient/ family. They may not understand the Medicare benefit and we would want to judiciously utilize the benefits that do exist.

Some Medicare members opt for an insurance company Medicare health plan. These plans follow Medicare guidelines but the insurance company requires authorizations for services. The insurance company may also contest medical necessity for a patient's inpatient hospital stay or rehab. Additionally, they may have limited providers in network. This can be a challenge to the case manager. Recommendations for a patient's discharge needs may not align with the insurance company's authorizations. This takes negotiation and compromise.

---

10   http;//www.Medicare.gov

"Some types of Medicare health plans that provide health care coverage aren't Medicare Advantage Plans but are still part of Medicare. Some of these plans provide: Medicare Part A (Hospital Insurance) and Medicare Part B (Medical Insurance) coverage, while most others provide only Part B coverage. Some also provide Medicare prescription drug coverage (Part D).

These plans have some of the same rules as Medicare Advantage Plans. However, each type of plan has special rules and exceptions"
Excerpt: http;//www.Medicare.gov

Rehab options need to be identified early on. In most hospitals the rehab team will make the evaluations and follow the patient, making rehab recommendations and identify goals.

Subacute rehab is generally a skilled level of care in a nursing home or a rehab center. It may also be utilized as a "swing bed" at some community hospitals. There needs to be a skilled need. E.g.: skilled physical therapy, occupational therapy, speech therapy. For Original Medicare the initial 20 days are covered if medically necessary. For managed care patients copays and coinsurance may vary. For Original Medicare days 21-100 of the SNF stay co-insurance is $167.50/ day. Days 101 and beyond are not covered. Always remember: observation hospital days do not count towards the 3 day inpatient qualifying days. The general rule of thumb is for an expected 1 hour of rehab daily. There is a social worker and an IDT at the SNF. The discharge plan needs to be established and communicated to the SNF prior to discharge.

People with Medicare are covered if they meet all of these conditions:

- *You have Part A and have days left in your benefit period.*
- *You have a qualifying hospital stay if you re-enter the same or another SNF within 30 days, you don't need another 3-day qualifying hospital stay to get additional SNF benefits. This is also true if you stop getting skilled care while in the SNF and then start getting skilled care again within 30 days.*
- *Your doctor has decided that you need daily skilled care given by, or under the direct supervision of, skilled nursing or therapy staff. If you're in the SNF for skilled rehabilitation services only, your care is considered daily care even if these therapy services are offered just 5 or 6 days a week, as long as you need and get the therapy services each day they're offered.*
- *You get these skilled services in a SNF that's certified by Medicare.*
- *You need these skilled services for a medical condition that was either:*
  - *A hospital-related medical condition.*
  - *A condition that started while you were getting care in the skilled nursing facility for a hospital-related medical condition.*

Excerpt: http;//www.Medicare.gov

If the patient is hospice eligible, sometimes an inpatient hospice facility is not always available. If the patient cannot have care provided at home, some families opt for hospice in a nursing home setting or group home setting. For longer term hospice patients there needs to be 2 payers: One for the SNF or group home and one for the hospice benefit. The other option would be for a designated hospice bed at a SNF which some hospices are able to do for a brief time. This varies by their contracts and policies. The SNF or group home may in fact be the patient's home. This option would support the patient dying in comfortable surroundings with hospice following the patient. Some SNFs bill the insurance and have a contract with the hospice. Some hospitals have the inpatient hospice contract with their local hospice. There may be minimal options, or may be several for the patient/ or family to choose from.

Acute rehab is generally for patients that can withstand 3-5 hours of rehab daily. It may include a wide interdisciplinary team, including a physiatrist (a physician that specializes in rehab). Again, the discharge plan needs to be identified. It is not always out of the question for a dying person to qualify and benefit from acute rehab. Nor is it a failure if the person would not be able to tolerate the acute rehab. Perhaps the patient might benefit from subacute rehab (if deemed appropriate) as a transition to maximize functional status.

I once had a male patient that was in excellent health prior to being ill. He was retired and active in his community. He began feeling progressively ill and he was admitted to the hospital. Findings were that he had extensive metastatic lung cancer. He was intubated due to bleeding in his lungs. An ethicist, an oncologist and the pulmonologist met with his family to set goals for his treatment. He was extubated and transferred to the medical floor. He underwent a swallow study. He was eventually able to tolerate foods orally, and the plan was to go home with hospice support. He had significant weakness, and would require extensive assistance getting out of bed. Care needs were anticipated to be around the clock. He made slow but steady progress and was deemed appropriate for an acute rehab stay.

I called after he was discharged home, where he was on hospice, and I found that his quality of life was excellent. He was able to get out of bed with a gait belt with stand by assistance. The family was instructed on transfers. He was eating for pleasure, even if in very small amounts, and was able to get out for daily rides looking at the fall foliage with his family. He talked with them and shared his innermost feelings. Best of all, he was able to feel independent and had dignity. He and his family were grateful to have had the time, the comfort, and the skills necessary to make it an optimal experience. They had the support of the hospice to deal with the dying process.

It can be very daunting to get what the patient may need. Don't reinvent the wheel.

Ask the patient if they have a prescription benefit. Some retirees have a "carve-out" supplemental insurance that is not simply a Medicare supplement policy. A secondary "carve-out" supplemental policy would act independently as a whole insurance policy, but would be billed only after the provider initially bills Medicare first. The "carve-out" polices vary by the employer. They may have a percentage for prescriptions, a tiered copay system for medications that may range from generic to higher specialty medications. They may have to have prior approval and/or justification that lower tier medications were tried and failed.

Some "carve-outs" have home infusion benefits, some do not.

If the patient is under 65, it can become more challenging. In order to access Medicaid, the patient needs to be deemed income eligible to qualify. If it is anticipated that the patient may be ill for months or indefinitely, they may be encouraged to apply for social security disability. It varies by institution. Some facilities use social workers to initiate disability and some use privately hired companies that specialize in this type of need. The patient needs to be disabled for 2 years or age 65 to qualify for Medicare. It is important to clarify the patient's goal, and what the anticipated disease progression is, and offer them options so as to help them make an informed decision. If the patient is young, married, or has school aged children, the goal may be to receive treatment and return to work as soon as possible. If the patient is the subscriber on the insurance policy, they may not want to do anything to jeopardize their ability to continue to work, or keep their insurance. If varies from company to company the amount of short term and/or long term disability that might be available for the employee.

If this same 45 year old has diffuse metastatic disease, then the options may be different. Perhaps this patient could take a short term disability. Some companies will keep a person on the payroll for an indefinite period of time, particularly small companies. In this case the decision might be different. If the patient has a spouse that could insure them, that might be an optimal solution. That is if it can be afforded and the spouse is eligible. Fortunately, we no longer have insurance company denials for pre-existing conditions as we did just a few years ago. It is wise to refer to social work, as the patient and family might be eligible for Medicaid, or other supports. In this case the social worker applied the patient for Medicaid as well as disability. It can be asked to expedite the Medicaid process, (or sometimes called AHCCCS) if there is need.

This interim time with little or no financial resources can be burdensome for the patient and/or family. Some patients may continue with a Cobra benefit under their employer. This is an employer mandate that is accessible for employees for up to 18 months after leaving the employer. It may be quite pricy- up to several hundred dollars a month- so even though it is an available option, it may be out of reach financially for many. In some states, Medicaid pays for the cobra payment or the actual insurance policy for this patient and/ or family. It is not a well-known fact, but it does happen. The Medicaid may pay for the copays, or may not, depending on the case.

At times patients may have a coagulopathy. They may require an anticoagulant therapy indefinitely. At over $100 a day, this may entail a huge expense for the patients, and is medically necessary. Anticoagulation therapy has many options today that were not available in past years. Many now have copay assistance programs or indigent programs.

Many injectable medications and other medications still require prior approval. If in doubt, it is best to call the patient's pharmacy first to ask them to "run" the medication. They are nearly always helpful to let us know if there is a co pay, how many doses are allowed, or if it is denied (usually requiring prior approval). The pharmacy can generally give the case manager the number to reach the prior approval pharmacy. Note: The pharmacy could be outsourced from the insurance company. Sometimes the approval time is 24-48 hrs. With a quick turn around this may be too late for the patient to be discharged. The case manager can ask to have it expedited on the phone, and usually this can be accomplished.

Some rural pharmacies do not carry injectable drugs or specialty medications. Make sure that they have it in stock before the patient is discharged. It is always good to anticipate any prior approvals early on in the patient's stay. If the patient is on IV vancomycin for instance, it is highly likely that they may need continued IV therapy at discharge, or the oral vancomycin which generally requires prior approval from the insurance company. If the patient is on anticoagulation therapy in the hospital, chances are they will require continued therapy at discharge, etc.

Often with "higher tiered" medications, prior approval is required. This is true particularly with some of the higher tier anti-inflammatory medications and some of the newer antiemetic drugs. Make sure that they are covered, and that there aren't limits on the amounts dispensed under the prior approval. This part of the discharge process can be time consuming for the case manager but it can help avert a problem for the patient after discharge.

E.g. A patient requires an antiemetic that is "higher tiered" and only a few pills a month are covered or ID (Infectious Disease) physician is recommending a specific antibiotic for discharge and the rehab will not accept as it is cost prohibitive. These are examples of barriers to discharge. Check with the medical team to clarify if there is another effective option first.

In the case of the 50+ year old single mom living with her son, his partner, and their newly born baby in rural Vermont, there were many barriers.

She had metastatic renal cancer, which required hospitalization for disease progression, pain and symptom management. She could not safely return home. The social worker in the community setting called to relay this and to share her safety concerns. The patient was alert and oriented, very ill, and essentially bed bound. I spoke with her urologist, who relayed that her condition was end-stage, and clarified that hospice would be the appropriate option. I met with the patient and offered her choices, and asked her what her goal was. She told me that she wanted to go to New Jersey. Her "family was all there", and that is where she really wanted to spend her last days. She told me that she felt like a burden to her son. She acknowledged that she had a clear understanding of her disease progression and what her options were. Chief barriers were identified: disability had not come through, and she was under 65 years old, so she could not get Medicare. If her goal was to go to New Jersey, she would need Medicaid in the state that she was going to, and the insurance would be problematic for the hospice agency providing care there. She had no money, no savings, and had not been able to work for quite some time. She was vulnerable, dependent, without options, and could not problem solve due to this along with her illness.

So what could we do? I brainstormed with my social worker. He called disability, but told me that it was taking too long. She was dying by the day, and we thought about what she should do. I called the main number for disability, and worked with the supervisor to expedite the patient's disability. I worked with the urologist to accomplish this as quickly as possible. I called the hospice in the area in New Jersey and spoke with their hospice director who listened to this patient's case presentation. We discussed the needs, barriers, and what was in the process. She told me that they would go ahead and set up the equipment and would accept this patient, even though there was no payer. She assured me that they would take care of her and her family in the end. We rallied funds to pay for a direct flight for her to go home and miraculously she made it there. I called a couple of days later. Hospice was in place, the patient and her family were at peace and her goal was accomplished. It took a lot of good people pulling together, but it was a very satisfying experience to accomplish this for this woman. She would have died alone in the hospital, but instead she was comfortable and had resolution.

"You should remember that though another may have more money, beauty, and brains than you, when it comes to the rarer spiritual values such as charity, self-sacrifice, honor, and nobility of heart, you have an equal chance with everyone to be the most beloved and honored of all people."

ARCHIBALD RUTLEDGE

Patients with anticipated disease progression may need a great deal of help. Many patients do not have the knowledge, strength, or resources to access them. It is important to not only think outside of the box, but to refer to any and all options available to the patient. If necessary, ask to brainstorm with someone that can help you. Ask if they have had a situation like this and what worked. Above all, don't give up trying.

I have been asked the question, "What if my insurance has lapsed? I was too sick to keep working, lost my job, and I am between coverage. Can my medical insurance be denied if I am sick?" This is a big concern for patients. Generally, if it is a small group policy there can be a lapse without any denial of coverage, and can no longer be denied for any pre-existing condition. Patients with a group insurance can have a 90 day break without loss in coverage. Non group insurance can have a 63 day break without loss of coverage.

"Non-group health insurance is insurance that you can buy on your own from an insurance company, instead of being part of a group (like at work). It's for both individuals and families. Anyone can buy non-group health insurance,

as long as they are not on Medicare or Medicaid. You can get non-group health insurance at any time, from most major insurance companies."[11]

The Affordable Care Act (ACA)

The comprehensive health care reform law enacted in March 2010 (sometimes known as ACA, PPACA, or "Obamacare").
The law has 3 primary goals:

- Make affordable health insurance available to more people. The law provides consumers with subsidies ("premium tax credits") that lower costs for households with incomes between 100% and 400% of the federal poverty level.
- Expand the Medicaid program to cover all adults with income below 138% of the federal poverty level. (Not all states have expanded their Medicaid programs.)
- Support innovative medical care delivery methods designed to lower the costs of health care generally.[12]

There has been much controversy and debate about the ACA, however most of us in healthcare see fewer and fewer uninsured patients today. Unfortunately out of pocket and copays may be quite high and contracted providers may be hard to find in some cases.

HIPAA

HIPAA- what does it mean? There has been a lot of talk about HIPAA and its implementation, but the focus is on patient

---

11   Health Care for All, 30 Winter Street, 10th floor, Boston, MA, 02108
12   www.affordable-health-insurance-plans.org/2018 Medicare.gov

protection and the protection of those rights:

> *"In enacting HIPAA, Congress mandated the establish-
> ment of federal standards for privacy of individually iden-
> tifiable health information. When it comes to personal
> information that moves across hospitals, doctors' offices, in-
> surers or third party payers, and State lines, our country has
> relied on a patchwork of federal and state laws. Under the
> patchwork of laws existing prior to adoption of HIPAA and
> the Privacy Rule, personal health information could be dis-
> tributed-without either notice or authorizations-for reasons
> that had nothing to do with a patient's medical treatment or
> health care reimbursement. For example, unless otherwise for-
> bidden by state or local law, without the Privacy Rule, patient
> information held by a health plan could, without the patient's
> permission, be passed on to a lender who could then deny the
> patient's application for a home mortgage or a credit card, or
> to an employer who could use it in personnel decisions. The
> Privacy Rule establishes a federal floor of safeguards to protect
> the confidentiality of medical information. State laws which
> provider stronger privacy protections will continue to apply
> over and above the new federal privacy standards. Health
> care providers have a strong tradition of safeguarding private
> health information. However, in today's world, the old system
> of paper records in locked filing cabinets is not enough. With
> information broadly held and transmitted electronically, the
> Rule provides clear standards for the protection of personal
> health information."[13]*

---

13   http;//www.hhs.gov/ocr/hipaa

If the patient is over 60, it is often advantageous to refer to your Area Agency on Aging. I always worked very closely with the AAA agencies when in home hospice and palliative care as well as in the inpatient setting for additional community resources. Their case managers are experts in accessing any and all resources in their community, including meals on wheels (MOW), Lifeline, long term Medicaid, volunteers, rides, and companionship services. These case managers are seasoned, strong patient advocates, and are a huge resource to our patients and families.

Home care, palliative care, hospice case managers, and social workers are equally important resources. Often the options can be initiated in the inpatient setting, with outpatient follow-up too. It is important to communicate what has been started and what the goals are. I would give the contact numbers to the patient and/or family to have readily available. Many times they are overwhelmed and can only absorb small pieces of the referrals. In time, usually once a patient returns home, it becomes more understandable. Never try to pull this together at discharge. I was told many years ago that, "Only 10% of what you say is retained at discharge, as the patient's head is already out the door." I have found this invaluable, and find that early case management contact, building of trust, and an ongoing relationship is the key.

Once again, ask the patient if he would like a referral to the insurance case manager if one is available. Unfortunately, insurance plans are complex and no two are alike. This can be very frustrating when setting up services for your patient. Some insurance companies have a case manager that follows the patient through the inpatient setting into the outpatient setting. The case manager would know the patient, have a working understanding of the insurance benefit, and would be the point person for coordination of care. Unfortunately, some companies outsource the case management, the durable medical equipment (DME), the ambulance, the home health, the hospice, etc., to different companies. This not only makes it confusing, but incredibly time consuming to coordinate needs after discharge. Try to record any and all contact names and numbers. Ask for any direct phone numbers or extensions if possible. Ask for any direct numbers that will minimize your wait time on hold or being transferred.

Some case management departments have set up clerical support to accomplish this, which is very helpful, but if there is no clerical support, or case management coordinators, try to make It as simple as you can. If you need an ambulance, find out what the restrictions are. Some companies only will allow emergent transfer of patients. Some may not be equipped for bariatric or special needs. If possible clarify as much in advance as you can. This can be quite a barrier if your patient was admitted via ambulance, but he or she cannot be transported home via car.

Medicare does not pay for patients to be transported via ambulance home. Some Medicaid plans pay for ambulance transfer or cabs based on the plan and needs. The patient and/or family may have to pay for the transport. If privately paying they would need to be offered a choice of at least 3 companies that could be utilized. Experience from peers or your own experience will give you a list of companies that are the most reasonable and provide quality care. It would be unfortunate to set it up only to find out that it isn't covered by the insurance and the patient and/or family is going to have to be billed several hundred dollars for the transport. Additionally, some insurance companies only contract with specific providers.

Ask the insurance case managers what the palliative or hospice plan would cover. I learned that one insurance company has only a $10,000 palliative and hospice benefit in total. We all know that that wouldn't last very long. If the patient needs palliative care, the hospice benefit would be exhausted before the patient could choose to access it. Under insurance case management the benefits can sometimes be flexed. Find out if it can. If not, let the patient/ family know so they can make choices. Some providers have limited palliative care services that can be offered. It is his/ her benefit, and the choice is his / hers.

If your insurance case manager does not know the patient's benefit, ask for the direct number to call so that you can find out. It isn't the optimal situation, but sometimes it is the best option that is available.

When meeting with your patient and/or family, know what the treatment options are and what the disease progression is. This is can often be approached during intradiciplinary rounds (IDT). Mostly, look at the patient. If this patient is dying, then ask the physician if hospice might be more appropriate. Do not underestimate this option for the patient. If it is clearly appropriate, then discuss this option with your patient and family after the physician(s) has addressed it with them.

IT IS IMPORTANT TO ACCESS THE
HOSPICE BENEFIT IF THE PATIENT:

- meets the criteria
- would benefit from the hospice benefit
- has a clear understanding of his/ her prognosis
- opts for the goal of comfort not cure

- opts for his/ her care in the hospice setting vs. in and out of the hospital
- would have better quality of life from the total package benefit of meds, equipment, volunteers

However, I tried to convey to my patients that it isn't appropriate if their goal isn't for pain and symptom management, or if for whatever reason they are not at "that place" philosophically, spiritually, or emotionally. In that case palliative care would be most appropriate. Let them process it, and then they can make it their decision. They may want to start out with palliative care and then transition to hospice if they choose. Always remember that our goal is to make the patient autonomous, not dependent. We may be thinking that this or that might be better, but we are not in their place. This is an all important thing to remember and practice.

End-Stage Disease and the Complexity it Presents

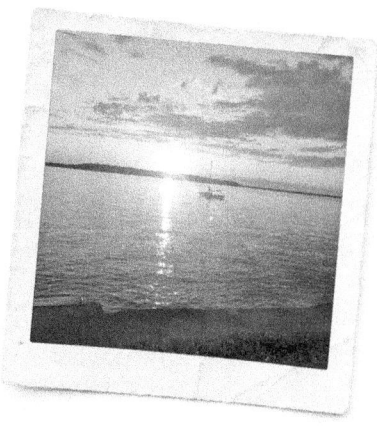

> *"And in the end, it's not the years in your life that count. It's the life in your years."*
>
> Abraham Lincoln

End-stage disease is one of the most challenging fields in case management. What does it mean and how do we handle these complicated patients? The definition of end-stage disease:

> *"The last phase in the course of a progressive disease. As in end-stage liver disease, end-stage lung disease, end-stage renal disease, end-stage cancer, etc. The term "end stage" has come to replace "terminal".*[14]

It really is no wonder why patients and families often don't grasp that their medical condition is a terminal condition. Even those of us in case management often have a hard time with

---

14   www.medicinenet.com

patients that are "end-stage". So many times we see these patients in and out of the hospital only to be re-admitted despite medical adherence, supports in place and best intentions. Should we approach these cases as chronic disease or would they be considered end-stage disease? This is the grey area that we can find ourselves in when approaching some of our patients and families.

In my last phase of my case management career, I worked in a 200 bed community hospital in Arizona. Much of my time was spent as an intensive care case manager. It is a floor based case management department so unless a patient is readmitted to the ICU, one might be unaware of their readmission. Additionally, the same patient might have several admits to various hospitals in the valley as well as rehab stays since their last admission.

Jacob was one of my patients that I would see come back in the hospital, usually critically ill. He was not diagnosed as end-stage, yet it was obvious that with each readmission he was becoming less functional; had longer stays; was unable to go directly home and required extensive rehab stays as a bridge to going home. He lived alone with his elderly wife who was very loving and devoted, but shared with me that she was becoming more exhausted and was unsure physically if she could meet her husband's needs. They had several children and their families, and they were very involved, however the bulk of the care was done by his wife. Jacob had home health services set up for additional support at home. Palliative care was consulted but palliative care was declined by the patient and his family. His goal was always to return home. His family would tell me "He's a fighter!" Home health services were arranged and time between admissions became closer and closer.

On his last admission to our hospital, Jacob was admitted to the ICU. He required mechanical ventilation, multiple drips and medications during this stay. His kidneys could no longer recover and he began inpatient dialysis for newly diagnosed end-stage renal disease(ESRD).

ESRD in itself is not considered a terminal diagnosis. Many patients go on to live functional lives in the community and undergo dialysis 3 times a week in the outpatient setting. There are a large number of patients that continue to work and may drive themselves to and from the dialysis center.

> *"The purpose of a doctor or any human in general should not be to simply delay the death of the patient, but to increase the person's quality of life."*
>
> PATCH ADAMS

What made Jacob different in this case was that he was so debilitated that he could no longer get out of bed even with extensive help. His dialysis would entail that he go to the outpatient dialysis center 3 times a week for several hours for each dialysis session. He was a high risk of readmission as well as high risk for re-intubation. He was not appropriate to go to SNF and he would not be able to tolerate going to an outpatient dialysis center. The discharge goal was to transition to an LTAC or a "high level SNF" (one that could manage his dialysis in house). Unfortunately, he had nearly exhausted his acute inpatient Medicare days as well as his SNF days. (He had not been out of the hospital or rehab setting for a 60 day period).

"Due to advancements in medical technology and management of illnesses such as sepsis, an increasing number of intensive care unit (ICU) patients are stabilized during acute illness following prolonged resuscitation and treatment. These patients develop metabolic, neuroendocrine, immunological, and neuromuscular disturbances, become dependent on intensive care therapies, and may require prolonged organ support. These patients are often described as being "chronically critically ill"(1). The development of this new type of patient in the modern era poses novel challenges for care, prognosis, and health care utilization in the ICU and after discharge"[15]

During IDT ICU rounding, input from the various disciplines was done. It was clarified with the intensivist, the palliative care physician, nursing and the therapy team that Jacob was no longer able to get out of bed despite multiple attempts. It was determined that he had multisystem organ failure. I was asked by our intensivist to meet with this family again to discuss the discharge barriers. The patient was very somnolent and was not able to participate. He was still in full code status, which meant that in the event of cardiopulmonary failure he and his family still wanted full life support. In the event that he could not breathe on his own this means that he would be re-intubated and receive cardiopulmonary resuscitation if needed. The team felt that this was contraindicated for this patient because of his advanced disease but he and his family did not want to change his "code status".

I met at length with Jacob's family, but it was not until I shared with them that the likelihood of Jacob returning home was not in

---

15   "Relationship Between ICU Length of Stay and Long-term Mortality for Elderly ICU Survivors"
https://www.ncbi.nlm.nih.gov/pubmed/26571190

the foreseeable future, did they begin to ask end of life questions. This all was despite multiple conversations with physicians with each readmission. The steadfast goal was for Jacob to return home and continue dialysis.

Jacob's wife was in shock as well as the entire family. They discussed with the ICU team that they did not want Jacob to be resuscitated or intubated if he worsened. The intensivist changed his code status to DNR/DNI. (Do Not Resuscitate/ Do Not Intubate). They insisted that I be with them and that he be told. I went with them to the bedside. Jacob was asleep but was awakened per his family's request. His goals were re-addressed. He was sleepy but alert. His condition deteriorated and his aggressive supports were withdrawn. He died peacefully with his family at his bedside.

> *"One-year mortality rate of long-term ICU-treated patient was 28 %, and this was predicted by age, disease severity, comorbidities and ICU re-admissions. The ICU survivors reported a lower IIRQL, and a minority of these patients returned home directly after hospital discharge; however, GPs reported numerous possible long-term complications."[16]*

As RN case managers we take our cues from the physician. Not all physicians have the expertise or comfort with end of life issues and this aspect of care. In his book, "Being Mortal", Dr. Atul Gawande addresses many individuals and the many aspects of the healthcare system. He speaks of these patents as they went from being independent, their aging and what it entailed, and their eventual death.

---

16   https://www.ncbi.nlm.nih.gov/pmc/articles/PMC4604105/

> *"Bob Arnold, a palliative care physician I'd met from the University of Pittsburgh, had explained to me that the mistake clinicians make in these situations is that they see their task as just supplying cognitive information- hard, cold facts and descriptions. They want Dr. Informative. But it's the meaning behind the information that people are looking for more than the facts. The best way to convey meaning is to tell people what the information means to you yourself, he said"*[17]

We can never assume that patients and families understand the prognosis and the choices. Often times it takes re-addressing goals of care by the admission, by the day or even by the hour. Once the prognosis is clear, it is vital to have the full family team meetings so that they can get input from all involved and make an informed decision. Families over the years have told me so many times that when a physician rounds, they hear from their specific perspective or component of the patient's illness. Another physician might be reported as telling the family their perspective. Patients and their families relay that they become confused and really don't fully understand what is going one.

Sometimes I suspect that because the patient may have had extensive hospital stays and/or readmissions they or their family may feel that they can be "fixed". After all, they have been in the past. Technology is so extensive now that there is usually a hope of recovery. When a person has CPR done on TV we might get the impression that the turn-around from such an event might be pretty uncomplicated. Unless the patient and family have experienced it themselves, they can be naive around what it might entail.

---

17   "Being Mortal" Atul Gawande

Palliative care input is vital in these complicated cases. It does not mean that all end of life patients want or should be hospice patients. It does mean that a palliative care physician or team would have the expertise and comfort with opening up the conversation. This would help ensure that we are addressing the patient's and families wishes, needs and goals in end of life situations.

Self Care

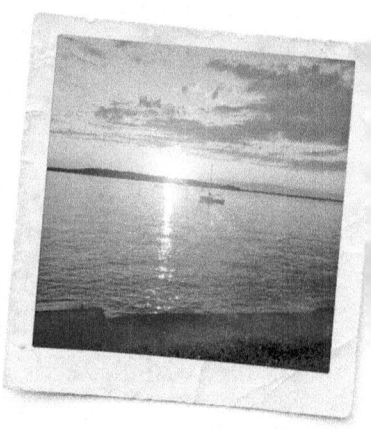

CHAPTER 6

> *"The best and most beautiful things in
> the world cannot be seen or even touched.
> They must be felt with the heart"*
>
> Helen Keller

SELF CARE-WHAT DOES IT MEAN? WHAT DOES IT MEAN TO A CASE MANAGER?

Self-**toward oneself**
Care- **regard**
Self Care= Regard towards oneself

We have always heard, "Be careful that you don't burn out." He or she is really "toasty". We used to hear, "Don't get attached. Don't show your emotions, it isn't professional."

Have you ever noticed that most of the same nurses that were doing end of life care fifteen or even twenty years ago are still going strong? I believe the reason for this is self-care. Taking care of ourselves is different for all of us. Whenever I see a lecture for continuing education regarding stress in the health care system, everybody lines up. We give so much of ourselves, and yet some of us find it nourishing and refreshing.

A while back one of my patients asked me "How can you do this all the time? You listen and hear so much pain and sadness, and yet you are always so happy?" My response was simple, and yet I have thought about it so many times since. When I look into the eyes of someone that I know may be dying, or is very ill, everything in that moment that was petty before, seems irrelevant. That is the truth. Things can be a flurry, and it doesn't mean that I haven't been all flustered at times, but generally I find it very balancing.

Some other things that I have learned over the years are:

SMILE

Seems kind of silly I know. But when you meet someone and smile, they will usually smile back. Patients have enough to deal with. They need a friendly face. Someone that they feel that they can trust and handle what they have to say. If you stand or sit there all tense, the patient probably won't feel comfortable sharing with you.

ENJOY THE SMALL THINGS

Over the years, we tend to look back on those small things and the way we felt. The way patients looked into your eyes, you felt like you could see their soul. The way their partner sat by their side, or the look on their face when their children or grandchildren hugged them. The way the nurse knew that they were really having a hard day and she gently put her hand on their shoulder. The way that special patient stayed up when she was so weak to make the fudge for the nurses and the doctors as a treat. The list goes on and on, but just look and you will see it.

TAKE EACH PATIENT VISIT AS A SEPARATE EXPERIENCE

This is one of the most valuable things that someone in hospice told me many years ago, and I have never forgotten it. Before I visit each patient, I try to stop for a minute and become centered. I try not to bring the experience from the previous patient to the next patient. Each patient is different, each life experience is different, and we learn from each and every one if we are open to it. It is much harder when it gets really busy, but if we greet one person at a time, the time goes quickly and we are present in the moment.

LISTEN TO YOUR INNER VOICE

I like to listen to music, or just daydream to unwind. Some days other things work, but I can always tell when I am not taking time for myself, because I can feel it inside. It may be different for each of us, but irritability, resentment, and fatigue are signs. We may think that we are too busy, but we need to self-nourish in a healthy way. If we just listen to that voice, we get the signal to slow down, take care of yourself, and it will help refocus you.

LAUGH, AND I MEAN REALLY LAUGH

Surround yourself with friends and people that make you feel good. Be with people that build you up. There is too much tearing down. The really silly belly laughing is the very best. You feel exhilarated after. Do it often and daily. Avoid the downers. It isn't good for us on a steady basis.

LAST BUT NOT LEAST, LOVE YOURSELF

Why is it that the Europeans have decadent chocolate and ice cream, and feel wonderful about it? I think that they are kinder to themselves, and feel that they deserve it. We should do more of that. Not beating ourselves for dessert, with all the calories, carbs, and fats. We should be at least as kind as we are to our patients, to OURSELVES on a routine basis. Give ourselves a pat on the back, and those around us that are doing so much as well.

It's contagious!

Patient Follow-Up and Companioning

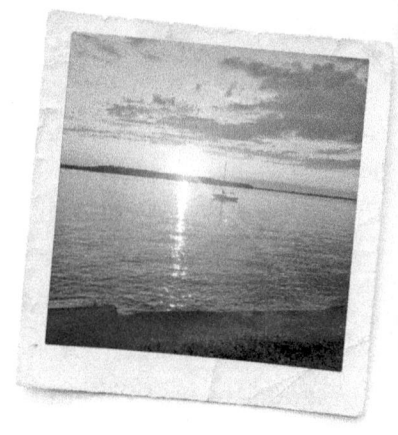

CHAPTER 7

"Angels can fly because they take themselves lightly"
G.K. CHESTERTON

There is a term that is used in hospice. It is called companioning of the patient. But what does that have to do with case management? That certainly is not a needed skill, you might say. I would offer that it is an essential component to good outcomes, patient support, and better quality of life for the patient and his or her family.

When a patient is admitted with a new diagnosis or a new metastatic lesion, it can be terrifying for them. A patient might be told that it can be cured, that radiation should take care of it, or that there are other viable options.

In the book *Final Gifts,* Maggie Callan and Patricia Kelly wrote:

"After exploring your feelings, try to imagine those of the dying person. By trying on the idea of dying you'll have a surer sense of what to say and how to help. At this point it's worth reflecting on the stages of dying as described by Dr. Kubler-Ross: denial, anger, bargaining, depression, acceptance.

Although Dr. Kubler-Ross has labeled these experiences "stages," a person doesn't necessarily progress through them in an orderly fashion. These emotions aren't exclusive to dying, either; any crisis or major life change can trigger them, which means that they will be familiar to almost any adult."[18]

As a case manager, I try to offer any and all options in the short time that I might see the patient in the hospital. The patient and family are offered choices, and then he or she can make informed choices regarding follow-up.

Perhaps as a case manager, you don't feel that there are a whole lot of options out there for your patient. You may feel that you don't feel that you could offer the person anything. Remember that sometimes small things are big things to our patients.

Years ago a case management colleague asked me to follow a 20 year old woman. She was married and had two small children. It was suspected that she had acute leukemia. She was admitted to her cardiology practice on telemetry with tachycardia and a newly diagnosed mediastinal mass. The case manager came to me feeling the acute pain of this young woman. The patient was close to the age of her own daughters. She said, "I think that you could offer her more." The patient was transferred to my oncology service, and I made the initial contact with patient, her spouse, and her family. She told me that they lived quite far away, and I listened

---

18   Final Gifts, Maggie Callanan and Patricia Kelley, 1992

to her story. I referred to my social work colleague for additional support and outpatient follow-up and I offered her many support options and lodging. The single most important support that she relayed later on was this: "I was so devastated, all I could do was break down and cry and cry. My husband and family were on the way, but the case manager just sat with me and held my hand. I don't know what I would have done without her." Sometimes the most important thing that we can do is exactly that, to just listen. We may not have to do anything for support. The patient may not want to hear another word from anyone. They may be too overwhelmed. They will always remember that someone took a minute to just listen. The rest can be set up when they can absorb it.

In palliative care and hospice, companioning is a key component. I would offer palliative care to as many of my metastatic cancer patients that I could. It can be a person or team that can follow them for pain and symptom management, be called if they have a question and be someone that is out there in the community to offer additional support. We have found that over the years support comes in many forms. It can be a phone call, or relationship that can be rallied in the event of need. It is much better to initiate the relationship early on and begin to set up services, then only to meet the patient and family at the so called "11th hour" when they don't know you and might feel anxious. We wouldn't want them to deal with that component when they are dealing with everything else.

Many clinics have social workers, and communities have a myriad of supports. Ask, share with your colleagues, and offer what you can. Allow the patient to decide what he would like to access.

It is good if you can follow-up with the patient or family

within a couple of days after discharge. I like to verify that pain and symptoms are being managed, answer questions, verify that home health, palliative care, or hospice has been initiated, and check on any other issues. Usually I have found that they are feeling well supported, and that services and equipment are in place. But occasionally, I find that pain could be out of control, that no one has been called, the caregiver is totally overwhelmed, or some other issue. In that situation a case manager can quickly avert a readmission, coordinate with the family, the provider(s), and the situation may quickly be turned around. Follow-up usually does not take but a few minutes, and almost always the patients or family will tell me that they really appreciated the call.

If follow-up calls are not part of your process, I would highly recommend it. You can start initially with your more complex patients that you have coordinated needs for and go from there. I have found that it is often one of the most rewarding pieces of my job.

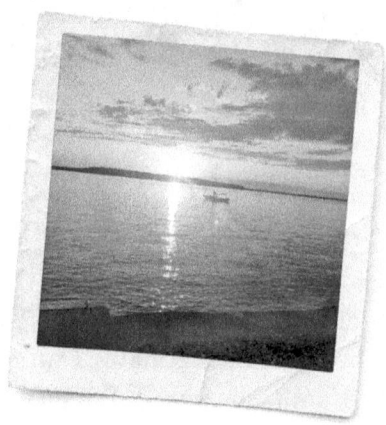

A Spiritual Journey

CHAPTER 8

"Out of every earth day, make a little bit of heaven."
ELLA WHEELER WILCOX

When many of us came into the nursing profession, we may have had high dreams of how it would be. Many of us looked for meaning in the baths that we gave, the medicines that we administered, and the technology that we needed to learn along the way. But for me, the most spiritual growth has to have come from being with the terminally ill and dying individuals. I use the word individuals because every young mother, every child, every grandfather all have touched my life in the most highly spiritual ways. Hospice is not all about death and dying. We tell our patients that it is also about quality of life, finding peace, and being comfortable physically, emotionally, and spiritually.

I have worked in end of life care: as a hospice and palliative care nurse, as an inpatient case manager, as an inpatient oncology case manager and late in my career as an ICU case manager.

Some of the patients were recently diagnosed, some had metastatic disease, some with end-stage disease, and some were nearing death. I tried to offer as much support that I could think of, and refer as many services as the patient or family would like. This would include social workers, palliative care clinicians or teams, and sometimes hospice. It is important to ask the patient what they would like and explain what might be offered for support. Again, many patients, families and staff do not understand what palliative care and hospice would offer, but it is significant. I cannot remember all the names of my patients, but I can remember all the faces and the look in their eyes. Sometimes I would see such sadness, and sometimes I would see such love and peace.

I always learn and continue to learn.

Palliative care and hospice are not just about death and dying. It is also not just about getting good pain and symptom management. It is supporting not only the patient, but also the family physically, spiritually and emotionally. Many have written wonderful books that have inspired us all. As time as evolved, many have been comfortable to share thoughts and feelings in end of life care. I have found this core of spirituality makes me want to continue and be near this ever growing process of supporting individuals, whether they choose to pursue aggressive treatment, or choose pain and symptom management with holistic support. If we are open to it, it can happen.

I once had a patient who had metastatic disease from head and neck cancer. His family was preparing to bring him home. He was admitted for spinal cord compression, with a very limited life expectancy. He was developing cognitive changes, and the family was asking how they would know if he was dying if he couldn't tell them. I knew that he was going to be followed by the hospice team upon arrival home and I knew that they would support not only this patient but his family. I told them that he would know when he was dying, because the dying patient is always the first one to know. Everyone in the hospice knows this, but families don't always know this. They need to be gently comforted.

Years ago, I had a patient that was from New Jersey. He had end-stage Parkinson's disease. He had lost his wife years before. His condition had deteriorated and he was admitted to a nursing home near his home. He had fallen and fractured his hip. His daughter told me that they were told that there was nothing more that could be done for him other than to make him comfortable. His only daughter lived in Vermont. She paid to have him flown home in a jet and took a leave of absence in order to care for him in his final days. He was cachectic, in a fetal position, and could no longer communicate verbally. Despite this, the young woman lovingly cared for her father and made him feel comfortable with hospice support. She told me that she wondered how she would know when he was actually dying, as he could never tell her. I told her that sometimes people leave signs, and that if we are open to them we might see them. We didn't talk about it again.

One morning she called the hospice and told us that her dad had died in the night. I went out to see her, and her father's body was already gone to the mortuary. She told me that she was soundly sleeping in the next room, when all of a sudden a brilliant light came into the room and she immediately got up. She said that she didn't feel afraid, but knew that it had somehow come from her dad. She went to his bedside. She told me that he had died peacefully without change or a pre warning, but she felt that his spirit had said good-bye. She was so comforted. As she told me about it, she told me that she had remembered our conversation on that earlier day.

A Spiritual Journey

"All I have seen teaches me to trust the
Creator for all that I have not seen."
RALPH WALDO EMERSON

One day I was driving out to see my hospice patient. His wife would always greet me. When she did, she was teary and experiencing significant anticipatory grief. The hospice social worker was supporting her husband, but also was supporting this patient's spouse. The patient was a wonderful man, was having a lot of pain, and was requiring daily visits to titrate his medications. It was effective, although he was becoming quite immobile. He was alert, talkative, and very interactive. His friends had done many household projects, were bringing in meals, and he was comfortable and at peace. One morning, like many mornings, I entered the basement and his wife greeted me as usual. When I entered the home, I felt an unexplainable feeling or aura. In that moment, I knew that this man was crossing into some other realm. I could physically feel it in the air. It was not scary, nor was there a visible sign of anything different in his condition. I felt it strongly, and have never felt anything like it since. I made my visit and affirmed that he was comfortable. We talked a bit, and he shared his peaceful thoughts. I left and received a call within a couple of hours. He had just simply died. There was no struggle. He just slipped away quite quickly, his wife told me.

Maggie Callanan and Patricia Kelley's book, "Final Gifts", had an effect on the hospice community by sharing about communication and awareness of the dying. Many individuals may report that it is very much like a dream like state.

One man that I followed in hospice many years ago was admitted to hospice at the very end of life, as many folks were in those days. We did not have palliative care in the earlier years. He had non-small lung cancer, and was having significant pain. He was a very private person and was very afraid of the pain. He was transitioned to a morphine subcutaneous infusion and was soon very comfortable. He was able to take rides with his wife, sit out in the back yard, or just visit, which he had not done for quite some time. Palliative and hospice nurses have expertise in pain and symptom management. We owe it to our patients to offer them this service early on, so that they never have to suffer needlessly. This man was not what many would consider a spiritual man. He was less fatigued, and would sit quietly with his wife talking with her about things that he didn't have the strength or energy to do earlier. One night, she said that he sat there and told her that he was dreaming that I came to see him, and that I was with a holy person. She did not stop him, but let him talk on. He told her that I held his hand, and handed his hand to the holy person. He said that I had told him that he was ok now; that he was alright; and that it was to ok to go. His wife told me that he closed his eyes, and that he died right there at that moment. He had been in pain, and was so afraid for so long that she told me that she was comforted by this, even with his physical loss.

A man with metastatic disease was a hospice patient. He was dearly loved by his wife and his children. He traveled all over the world in his lifetime and loved to sail. As his condition worsened he became less responsive. When he was more responsive he told us a story. He said that he sailed in his dream. He told us that he would first go around a little island. He would then go ashore and find a table with his favorite donuts. Each day he would share that he would go a little farther, and a table would be filled with his favorite donuts, pastries and treats that he had always loved. Each day he would be more and more reluctant to "come back". He told his family this. Finally, one day he told them his experience, and they told him that he didn't have to come back, and that it was ok if he was happy. Each day he became less responsive, and finally slipped into death quietly.

"How silently, how silently, the wondrous gift is given."
PHILLIPS BROOKS

If your patient wants to go home, if the disease is in its end-stage, as a case manager, it is so important to help honor the patient's wishes. Sometimes patients choose to continue to fight in hope of slowing of the disease, but if the patient wants to go home, we need to speak with the team and help facilitate this.

One of the dearest women that I have ever met was from a large city. She was a highly successful professional woman that had tried many treatment options, but the disease continued to progress throughout treatment. She wanted to come to Vermont to be with her grown daughter and family. The other grown children came to Vermont to spend the last days with her. She was very swollen, very weak, and had been suffering significant pain. Her goal was to be with her family to say what she wanted to say, and to be surrounded by them. Her pain was at a very high level, and she told me that she had been enduring it for quite some time.

I received a call from my hospice director near the end of the day. This woman was having significant breakthrough pain that was rapidly escalating. I remember helping her into her nightgown, guiding her swollen, weak body onto the commode, and helping her into bed. I had stopped on my way home from work to start a morphine infusion, because when I had stopped earlier she was not getting adequate pain relief. There was also a question of analgesic absorption. I started her infusion, and she said to me, "Thank you. Now I can go." I have never forgotten those words, the way she looked, or the way that I felt during this experience at the end of a long day. It was beautiful.

The family told me that they all poured a drink and said a toast to honor their mom. She was slipping into unconsciousness. They told me that they knew that she was still aware that they were with her; and that she raised her arm up in recognition of their toast. She then died.

As case management grows across this country, and as palliative care and hospice grow also, I would encourage each case manager to get to know his or her local palliative care and hospice. Read more about the subject, prepare your own advanced directive, or maybe volunteer a small amount of your time each month. I guarantee that you will get more out of it than you will give. We owe it to our patients to offer the very best in end of life care.

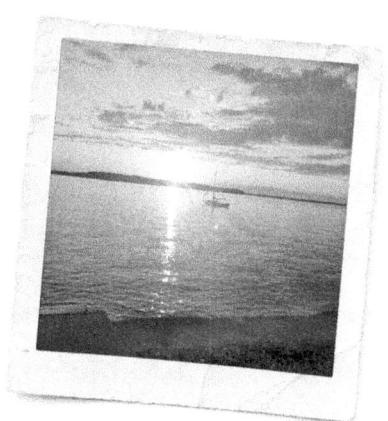

Conclusion

"Life is eternal; and love is immortal; and
death is only a horizon; and a horizon is
nothing save the limit of our sight."
ROSSITER WORTHINGTON RAYMOND
1840-1918 *Final Gifts*

We have more insight now into the dying process. We know what works and what doesn't work so well. Each individual is unique. We could spend hours talking about the experiences that we have had in nursing, in hospice, and in case management. We could laugh or cry, and sometimes our heart swells remembering the person or experience.

My words of wisdom are not new, nor are they complicated. Be present with the patient, and have courage and faith that you can be of help. For without you they might have nothing. Don't feel like you have to say the right things. Listen to your heart, and it will come with experience and patience.

The medical system is complex and often difficult for patients and for us as well. Working together helps.

Sometimes taking a break, getting input, and then re-looking at the barriers helps.

Remember to not just look at the task. Be aware of the holistic needs of our patients, and do what you can do. It is better than doing nothing. Try to always see things from the patient's perspective.

Stay centered, take care of yourself, be happy, and find joy in life.

> *"We've been wrong about what our job is in medicine. We think our job is to ensure health and survival. But really it is larger than that. It is to enable well-being."*
>
> ATUL GAWANDE

References/ Web Sites/ and Suggested Readings

American Academy of Family Physicians, Copy right 2004

American Pain Society, Principles of Analgesic Use in the Treatment of Acute Pain and Cancer Pain, 4th ed, Glenview, Ill. Author; 1999

Callanan, Maggie and Kelley, Patricia "Final Gifts" 1992

CMSA.org- Case Management Society of America

Gawande, Atul "Being Mortal: Illness, Medicine and What Matters in the End"

The Department of Health and Human Services (HHS) http://www.hhs.gove/ocr/hipaa

HPNA.org-Hospice and Palliative Nurses Association

http;//www.Medicare.gov

Hospice Standards of Practice, National

Hospice and Palliative Care Organization <http;//www.nhpco. org.2000.

"Journal of Hospice and Palliative Nursing" Vol.6, NO1, January- March 2004

Hospice Foundation of America

Last Acts, 1997

Pagels, Douglas Editor "May You Always Have an Angel by Your Side" 2001

Kubler-Ross, Elizabeth "On Death and Dying" 1969

www.ingramcontent.com/pod-product-compliance
Lightning Source LLC
Chambersburg PA
CBHW051345170526
45166CB00002B/974